MW01016570

THE ESSENTIAL VEGETARIAN KETO COOKBOOK

50 Hand-Picked Vegetarian Recipes for a
Healthy Keto Diet Lifestyle.

ISABELLA TAYLOR

TABLE OF CONTENTS

—

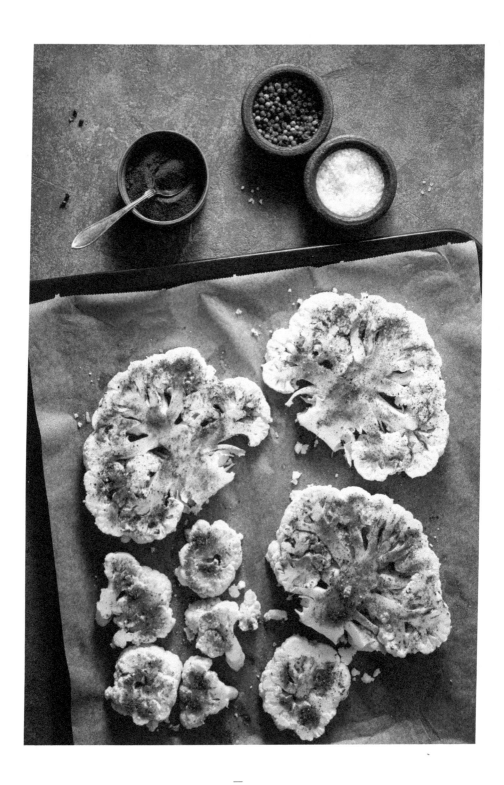

GUILT FREE LEMON AND ROSEMARY DRINK

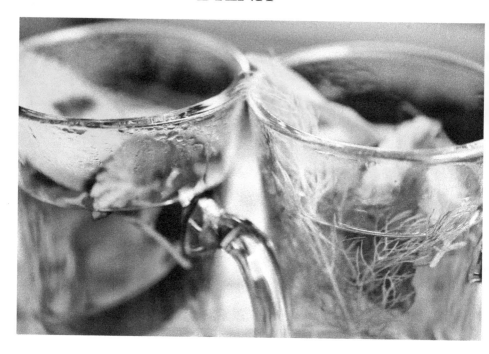

Serving: 1

Prep Time: 10 minutes

Ingredients:

- ½ cup whole milk yogurt
- 1 cup Garden greens
- 1 pack stevia
- 1 tablespoon olive oil
- 1 stalk fresh rosemary
- 1 tablespoon lemon juice, fresh

- 1 tablespoon pepitas

- 1 tablespoon flaxseed, ground

- 1 and ½ cups water

Directions:

1. Add listed ingredients to blender

2. Blend until you have a smooth and creamy texture

3. Serve chilled and enjoy!

Nutritional Contents:

- Calories: 312

- Fat: 25g

- Carbohydrates: 14g

- Protein: 9g

CREAMY LEEKS PLATTER

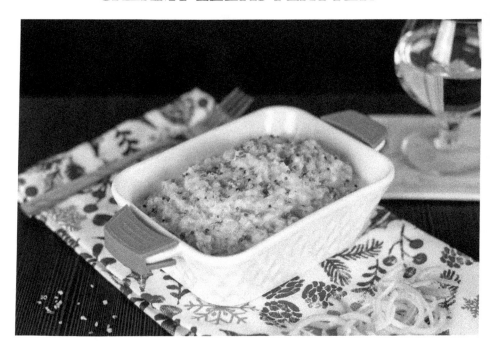

Serving: 6

Prep Time: 10 minutes

Cook Time: 25 minutes

Ingredients

- 1 and ½ pound leaks, trimmed and chopped into 4 inch pieces
- 2 ounces butter
- 1 cup coconut cream
- 3 and ½ ounces cheddar cheese
- Salt and pepper to taste

Directions

1. Pre-heat your oven to 400-degree F

2. Take a skillet and place it over medium heat, add butter and let it heat up

3. Add leeks and Sauté for 5 minutes

4. Spread leeks in greased baking dish

5. Boil cream in saucepan and lower heat to low

6. Stir in cheese, salt and pepper

7. Pour sauce over leeks

8. Bake for 15-20 minutes and serve warm

9. Enjoy!

Nutrition (Per Serving)

- Calories: 204
- Fat: 15g
- Carbohydrates: 9g
- Protein: 7g

CHEESY BROCCOLI AND CAULIFLOWER

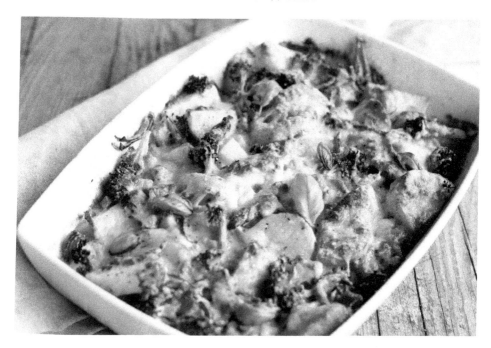

Serving: 4

Prep Time: 10 minutes

Cook Time: 10 minutes

<u>Ingredients</u>

- 1 pound broccoli, chopped
- 2 ounces butter
- 8 ounces cauliflower, chopped
- 5 and 1/3 ounces shredded cheese
- Salt and pepper , to taste

- 4 teaspoons sour cream

Directions

1. Take a large skillet and melt butter
2. Stir in all the vegetables
3. Sauté until it turns into golden brown over medium-high heat
4. Add all the remaining ingredients to the vegetable
5. Mix well
6. Serve warm and enjoy!

Nutrition (Per Serving)

- Calories: 244
- Fat: 20.5g
- Carbohydrates: 3.4g
- Protein: 12.2g

DASHING BOK CHOY SAMBA

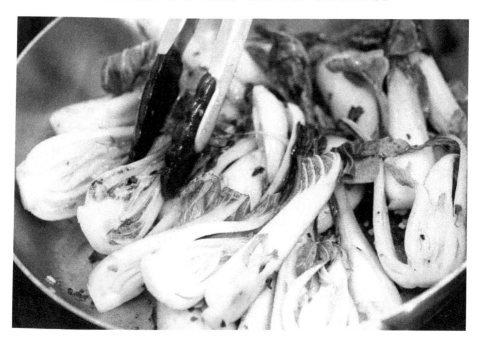

Serving: 3

Prep Time: 5 minutes

Cook Time: 15 minutes

<u>Ingredients</u>

- 4 bok choy , sliced
- 1 onion, sliced
- ½ cup Parmesan cheese, grated
- 4 teaspoons coconut cream
- Salt and freshly ground black pepper , to taste

Directions

1. Mix bok choy with black pepper and salt

2. Take a cooking pan, heat the oil and onion slice to sauté for 5 minutes

3. Then add cream and seasoned bok choy

4. Cook for 6 minutes

5. Stir in Parmesan cheese and cover the lid

6. Reduce the heat to low and cook for 3 minutes

7. Serve warm and enjoy!

Nutrition (Per Serving)

- Calories: 112
- Fat: 4.9g
- Carbohydrates: 1.9g
- Protein: 3g

TENDER COCONUT AND CAULIFLOWER RICE WITH CHILI

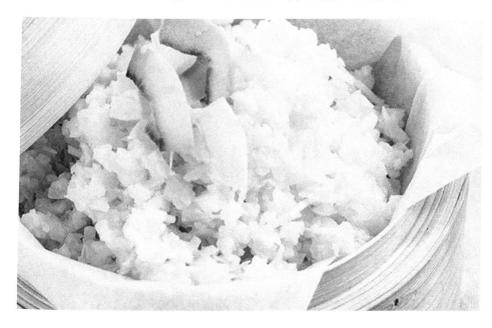

Serving: 4

Prep Time: 20 minutes

Cook Time: 20 minutes

Ingredients

- 3 cups cauliflower, riced
- 2/3 cups full-fat coconut milk
- 1-2 teaspoons sriracha paste
- ¼- ½ teaspoon onion powder
- Salt as needed
- Fresh basil for garnish

Directions

1. Take a pan and place it over medium low heat

2. Add all of the ingredients and stir them until fully combined

3. Cook for about 5-10 minutes, making sure that the lid is on

4. Remove the lid and keep cooking until any excess liquid goes away

5. Once the rice is soft and creamy, enjoy!

Nutrition (Per Serving)

- Calories: 95
- Fat: 7g
- Carbohydrates: 4g
- Protein: 1g

COOL ASPARAGUS TART

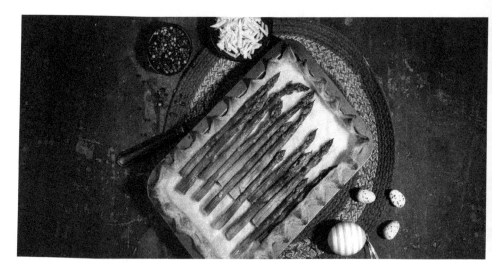

Serving: 4

Prep Time: 10 minutes

Cook Time: 20 minutes

Ingredients

- 4 whole eggs
- 1 garlic clove, chopped
- Salt and pepper to taste
- 20 asparagus spears, woody ends removed
- ½ cup cheddar cheese, grated
- 2 tablespoons walnuts, chopped

Directions

1. Pre-heat your oven to 375 degree F

2. Grease a pie dish with butter

3. Place eggs, garlic, pepper and salt to a small bowl and beat using fork

4. Pour egg mix into your tray

5. Lay asparagus onto egg into one row

6. Sprinkle grated cheese over asparagus

7. Place in oven and cook for 12 minutes until cheese melts

8. Enjoy!

Nutrition (Per Serving)

- Calories: 160

- Fat: 10g

- Carbohydrates: 5g

- Protein: 12g

SUCCULENT CHEESY CAULIFLOWERS

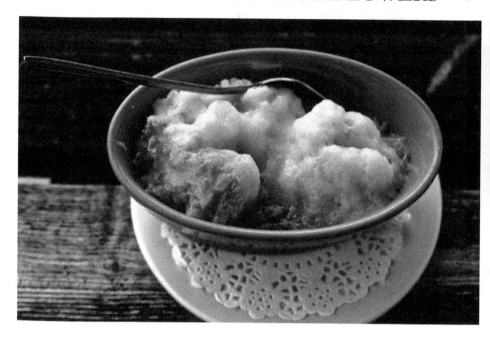

Serving: 3

Prep Time: 10 minutes

Cook Time: 25 minutes

Ingredients

- 1 cauliflower head
- ¼ cup butter, cut into small pieces
- 1 teaspoon Keto –Friendly Mayo
- 1 tablespoon Keto-Friendly Mustard
- ½ cup parmesan cheese, grated

Directions

1. Pre-heat your oven to 390 degree F
2. Add mayo and mustard in a bowl
3. Add cauliflower to mayo mix and toss
4. Spread cauliflower in baking dish and top with butter
5. Sprinkle cheese on top
6. Bake for 25 minutes
7. Serve and enjoy!

Nutrition (Per Serving)

- Calories: 228
- Fat: 20g
- Carbohydrates: 6g
- Protein: 3g

CREAMY CAULI MUSHROOM RISOTTO

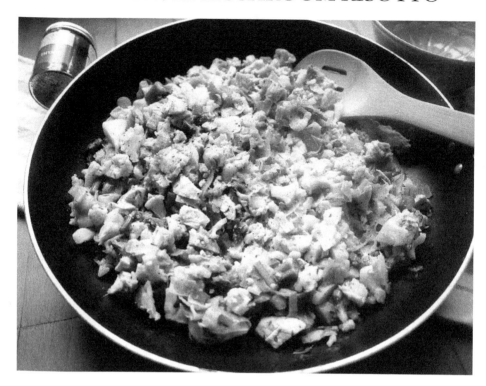

Serving: 4

Prep Time: 10 minutes

Cook Time: 20 minutes

Ingredients

- 1 cup vegetable stock
- 1 head of cauliflower, grated
- 9 ounces mushroom, chopped
- 2 tablespoons butter
- Salt and black pepper , to taste

- 1 cup coconut cream

Directions

1. Take a saucepan and pour stock into it
2. Bring it to boil and set it aside
3. Then take a skillet and melt butter over medium heat
4. Add mushroom to sauté until it turn into golden brown
5. Stir in a stock and grated cauliflower
6. Bring the mixture to a simmer and add cream
7. Cook until liquid is reduced and cauliflower is aldente
8. Serve warm and enjoy!

Nutrition (Per Serving)

- Calories: 186
- Fat: 16.5g
- Carbohydrates: 6.7g
- Protein: 2.8g

HEARTY GREEN BEAN ROAST

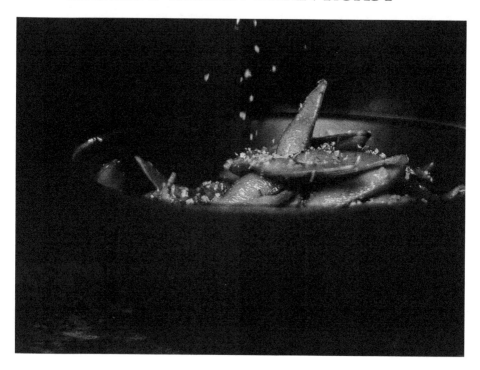

Serving: 4

Prep Time: 10 minutes

Cook Time: 20 minutes

Ingredients

- 1 whole egg
- 2 tablespoons olive oil
- Salt and pepper to taste
- 1 pound fresh green beans
- 5 and ½ tablespoons grated parmesan cheese

Directions

1. Pre-heat your oven to 400 degree F

2. Take a bowl and whisk in eggs with oil and spices

3. Add beans and mix well

4. Stir in parmesan cheese and pour the mix into baking pan (lined with parchment paper)

5. Bake for 15-20 minutes

6. Serve warm and enjoy!

Nutrition (Per Serving)

- Calories: 216
- Fat: 21g
- Carbohydrates: 7g
- Protein: 9g

ALMOND AND BLISTERED BEANS

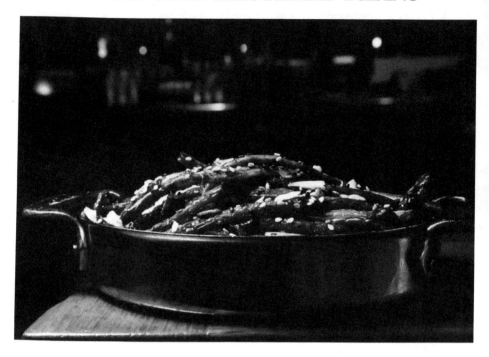

Serving: 4

Prep Time: 10 minutes

Cook Time: 20 minutes

Ingredients

- 1 pound fresh green beans, ends trimmed
- 1 and ½ tablespoon olive oil
- ¼ teaspoon salt
- 1 and ½ tablespoons fresh dill, minced
- Juice of 1 lemon
- ¼ cup crushed almonds

- Salt as needed

Directions

1. Pre-heat your oven to 400 degree F

2. Add in the green beans with your olive oil and also with salt

3. Then spread them in one single layer on a large sized sheet pan

4. Roast it up for 10 minutes and stir it nicely, then roast for another 8-10 minutes

5. Remove it from the oven and keep stirring in the lemon juice alongside the dill

6. Top it up with crushed almonds and some flak sea salt and serve

Nutrition (Per Serving)

- Calories: 347
- Fat: 16g
- Carbohydrates: 6g
- Protein: 45g

CHIPOTLE KALE CHIPS

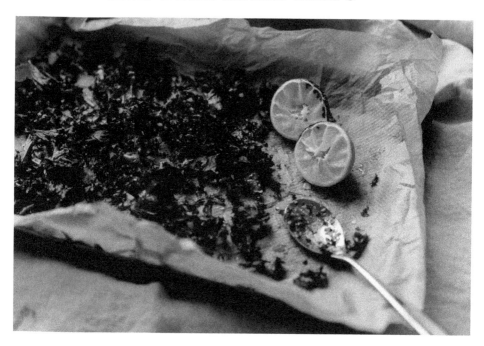

Serving: 4

Prep Time: 4 minutes

Cook Time: 29 minutes

Ingredients

- 2 large bunch kale, chopped into 4 pieces and stemmed
- 1 tablespoon olive oil
- 1/8 teaspoon salt
- 1 teaspoon chipotle powder
- ¼ cup parmesan cheese, shredded

Directions

1. Wash kale thoroughly and dry, cut into 4 inch pieces
2. Pre-heat your oven to 250 degree F
3. Take a baking sheet and line with parchment paper
4. Take a bowl and add kale, coat the kale with olive oil, chipotle and cheese
5. Transfer the mix to baking sheet
6. Bake for 19 minutes and check the crispiness
7. If you need more crispiness, bake for 9 minutes more
8. Serve and enjoy!

Nutrition (Per Serving)

- Calories: 37
- Fat: 3g
- Carbohydrates: 2g
- Protein: 1g

CLASSIC GUACAMOLE

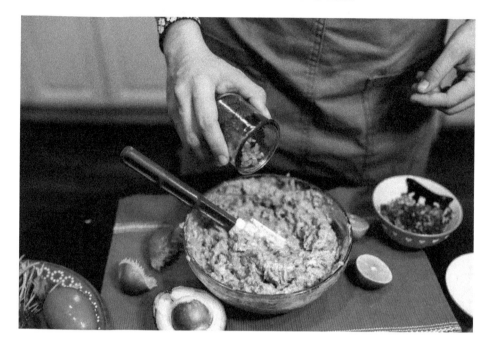

Serving: 6

Prep Time: 15 minutes

Cook Time: Nil

Ingredients

- 3 large ripe avocados
- 1 large red onion, peeled and diced
- 4 tablespoon of freshly squeeze lime juice
- Salt as needed
- Freshly ground black pepper as needed
- Cayenne pepper as needed

Directions

1. Halve the avocados and discard stone

2. Scoop flesh from 3 avocado halves and transfer to a large bowl

3. Mash using fork

4. Add 2 tablespoon of lime juice and mix

5. Dice the remaining avocado flesh (remaining half) and transfer to another bowl

6. Add remaining juice and toss

7. Add diced flesh with the mashed flesh and mix

8. Add chopped onions and toss

9. Season with salt, pepper and cayenne pepper

10. Serve and enjoy!

Nutrition (Per Serving)

- Calories: 172
- Fat: 15g
- Carbohydrates: 11g
- Protein: 2g

ASTONISHINGLY SIMPLE LETTUCE SALAD

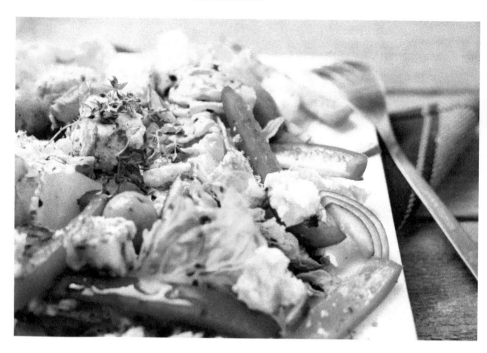

Serving: 2

Prep Time: 10 minutes

Cook Time: Nil minutes

Ingredients

- 2 ounces Romaine lettuce
- ½ ounce butter
- 1 ounce Adam cheese, sliced
- ½ avocado, sliced
- 1 cherry tomato, sliced

- 1 red bell pepper, sliced

Directions

1. Add butter on top of each lettuce leaves

2. Add alternating layers of cheese, avocado, tomato slices

3. Serve and enjoy!

Nutrition (Per Serving)

- Calories: 104

- Fat: 14g

- Carbohydrates: 4g

- Protein: 4g

LIGHT EGG SALAD

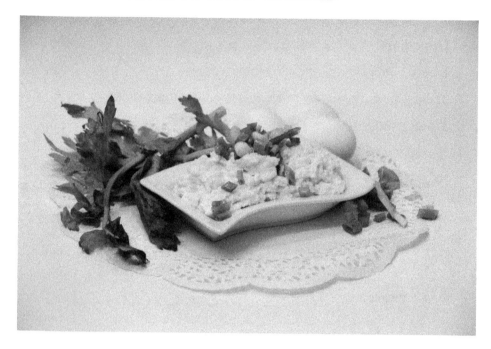

Serving: 4

Prep Time: 5 minutes

Cook Time: 15 minutes

Ingredients

- 3 hard-boiled eggs, cooled
- 2 tablepoons celery, diced
- 3 tablespoon canned coconut milk
- 1 tablesooon parsley, chopped
- 1 teaspoon fresh lemon juice
- Salt and pepper as needed

- 1 and ½ cups romain lettuce, chopped

Directions

1. Peel eggs and chop them coarsely, transfer to your salad bowl

2. Add celery, coconut milk, parsley, lemon juice and season with salt and pepper according to your taste

3. Sprinkle chopped romaine lettuce

4. Serve and enjoy!

Nutrition (Per Serving)

- Calories: 300
- Fat: 24g
- Carbohydrates: 3g
- Protein: 18g

BUTTERY GREEN CABBAGE

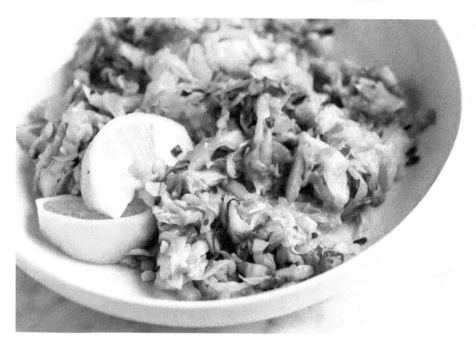

Serving: 4

Prep Time: 10 minutes

Cook Time: 15 minutes

<u>Ingredients</u>

- 1 and ½ pounds shredded green cabbage
- 3 ounces butter
- Salt and pepper to taste
- 1 dollop, whipped cream

Directions

1. Take a large skillet and place it over medium heat

2. Add butter and melt

3. Stir in cabbage and Saute for 15 minutes

4. Season accordingly

5. Serve with a dollop of cream

6. Enjoy!

Nutrition (Per Serving)

- Calories: 199

- Fat: 17g

- Carbohydrates: 10g

- Protein: 3g

THE GREAT CABBAGE SLAW

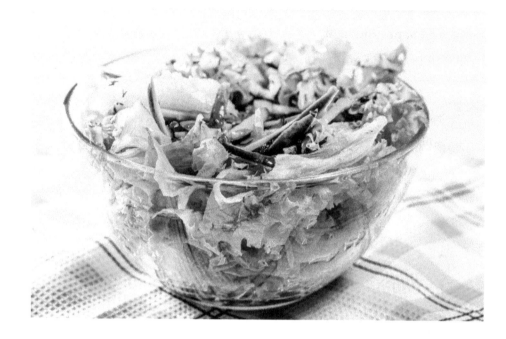

Serving: 6

Prep Time: 10 minutes

Cook Time: Nil

Ingredients

- 12 ounces green and red cabbage, shredded and mixed
- 4 ounces kale, chopped
- 1 cup Keto-Friendly mayonnaise
- ½ teaspoon each salt and pepper

Directions

1. Add listed ingredients to a bowl and mix well using spatula

2. Serve immediately or chilled

3. Enjoy!

Nutrition (Per Serving)

- Calories: 266
- Fat: 26g
- Carbohydrates: 6g
- Protein: 0.6g

AMAZING GREEN CREAMY CABBAGE

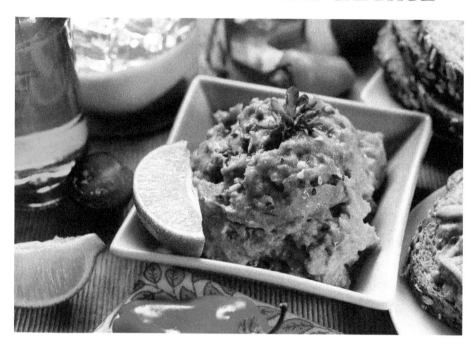

Serving: 4

Prep Time: 10 minutes

Cook Time: 10 minutes

Ingredients

- 2 ounces butter
- 1 and ½ pounds green cabbage, shredded
- 1 and ¼ cups coconut cream
- Salt and pepper to taste
- 8 tablespoons fresh parsley, chopped

Directions

1. Take a skillet and place it over medium, add butter and let it melt

2. Add cabbage and Saute until browns

3. Stir in cream and lower down the heat to low

4. Let it simmer

5. Season with salt and pepper

6. Garnish with parsley and serve

7. Enjoy!

Nutrition (Per Serving)

- Calories: 432
- Fat: 42g
- Carbohydrates: 8g
- Protein: 4g

PORTOBELLO MUSHROOM RISOTTO

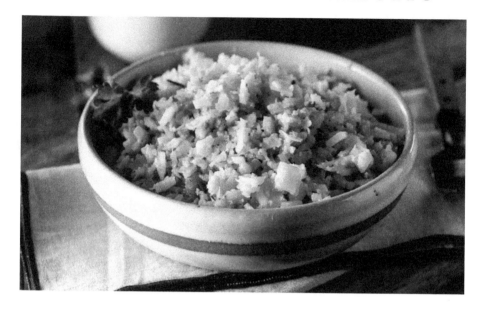

Serving: 4

Prep Time: 5 minutes

Cook Time: 15 minutes

Ingredients

- 4 and ½ cups cauliflower, riced
- 3 tablespoons coconut oil
- 1 pound Portobello mushrooms, thinly sliced
- 1 pound white mushrooms, thinly sliced
- 2 shallots, diced
- ¼ cup organic vegetable broth
- Salt and pepper to taste
- 3 tablespoons chives, chopped

- 4 tablespoons butter
- ½ cup parmesan cheese, grated

Directions

1. Use a food processor and pulse cauliflower florets until riced
2. Take a large saucepan and heat up 2 tablespoons oil over medium-high flame
3. Add mushrooms and Saute for 3 minutes until mushrooms are tender
4. Clear saucepan of mushrooms and liquid and keep them on the side
5. Add rest of the 1 tablespoons oil to skillet
6. Toss shallots and cook for 60 seconds
7. Add cauliflower rice, stir for 2 minutes until coated with oil
8. Add broth to riced cauliflower and stir for 5 minutes
9. Remove pot from heat and mix in mushrooms and liquid
10. Add chives, butter, parmesan cheese
11. Season with salt and pepper
12. Serve and enjoy!

Nutrition (Per Serving)

- Calories: 438
- Fat: 17g
- Carbohydrates: 15g
- Protein: 12g

GRIPPING EGGPLANT PARMESAN

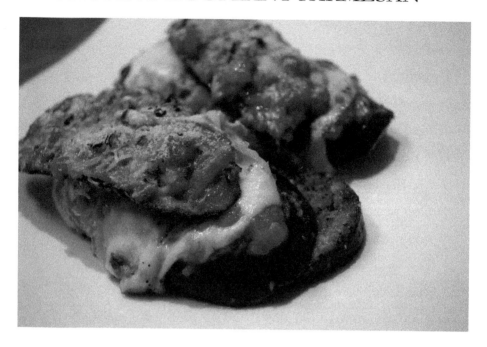

Serving: 2

Prep Time: 15 minutes

Cook Time: 6 minutes

Ingredients

- 1 medium eggplant
- ½ teaspoon salt
- 1 large egg
- 1 cup almond flour
- 1 cup parmesan cheese, grated
- 2 teaspoon garlic powder
- Salt and pepper to taste

- ¼ cup coconut oil

Directions

1. Prepare eggplant by slicing it into thin slices
2. Lay slices on a flat surface and blot with hand towel to remove excess water
3. Season with salt and pepper
4. Let it marinate for 30 minutes
5. Blot once more
6. Add eggs to a medium bowl and whisk
7. Add garlic powder, parmesan cheese, almond flour to a large bowl and season with salt and pepper, stir well
8. Place a skillet over medium heat and add coconut oil
9. Add eggplant slices to egg bowl and dredge them flour mix
10. Life out and add to hot oil
11. Fry until both sides are golden
12. Repeat until all eggplants are cooked
13. Enjoy!

Nutrition (Per Serving)

- Calories: 271
- Fat: 22g
- Carbohydrates: 10g
- Protein: 12g

THE RUTABAGA WEDGE DISH

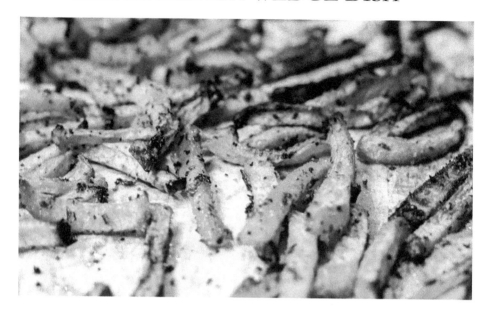

Serving: 4

Prep Time: 15 minutes

Cook Time: 45 minutes

Ingredients

- 2 medium rutabagas, medium, cleaned and peeled
- 4 tablespoons butter
- ½ teaspoon salt
- ½ teaspoon onion powder
- 1/8 teaspoon black pepper
- ½ cup buffalo wing sauce
- ¼ cup blue cheese dressing
- 2 green onions, chopped

Directions

1. Pre-heat your oven to 400 degree F

2. Line a baking sheet with parchment paper

3. Wash and peel rutabagas, clean and peel them and cut into wedge shapes

4. Take a skillet and place it over low heat, add butter and melt

5. Stir in onion powder, salt, onion, black pepper

6. Use seasoned butter to coat wedges

7. Arrange wedges in a single layer on baking sheet

8. Bake for 30 minutes

9. Remove and coat in buffalo sauce and return to oven

10. Bake for 15 minutes more

11. Place wedges on serving plate and trickle with blue cheese dressing

12. Garnish with chopped green onion and enjoy!

Nutrition (Per Serving)

- Calories: 235
- Fat: 15g
- Carbohydrates: 10g
- Protein: 2.5g

CREATIVE LEMON AND BROCCOLI DISH

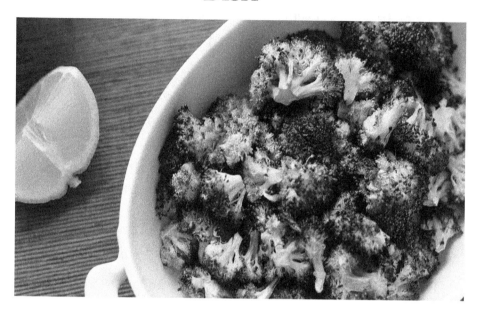

Serving: 6

Prep Time: 10 minutes

Cook Time: 15 minutes

Ingredients

- 2 heads brococli, separated into florets
- 2 teaspoons extra virgin olive oil
- 1 teaspoon salt
- ½ teaspoon black pepper
- 1 garlic clove, minced
- ½ teaspoon lemon juice

Directions

1. Pre-heat your oven to 400 degree F

2. Take a large sized bowl and add broccoli florets

3. Drizzle olive oil and season with pepper, salt and garlic

4. Spread broccoli out in single even layer on a baking sheet

5. Bake for 15-20 minutes until fork tender

6. Squeeze lemon juice on top

7. Serve and enjoy!

Nutrition (Per Serving)

- Calories: 49
- Fat: 1.9g
- Carbohydrates: 7g
- Protein: 3g

SPINACH AND TOMATO ZOODLES

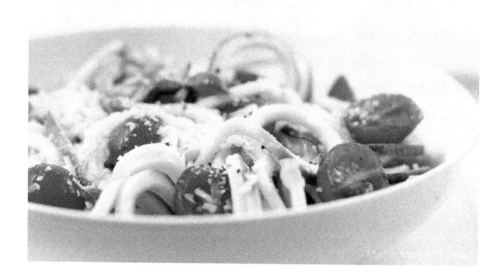

Serving: 4

Prep Time: 10 minutes

Cook Time: 10 minutes

Ingredients

- 3 tablespoons olive oil

- 1 tablespoon butter

- $1^1/2$ tablespoons minced garlic

- 1 cup packed fresh spinach

- $^1/2$ cup halved cherry tomatoes

- 2 tablespoons chopped fresh basil $^1/2$ cup sliced black olives

- 3 zucchinis, spiralized

- $^1/2$ cup shredded Asiago cheese
- Sea salt and freshly ground black pepper, to taste

Directions

1. In a nonstick skillet, heat the olive oil and melt the butter over medium-high heat. Add and saute the garlic for 2 minutes or until fragrant.

2. Add and saute the spinach, tomatoes, basil, and olives for 4 minutes or until the spinach wilts, then add the spiralized zucchini and toss with a fork to coat well. Scatter with Asiago cheese and cook for 2 minutes or until the zucchini is soft and the cheese melts.

3. Sprinkle with salt and ground black pepper. Remove them from the

Nutrition (Per Serving)

- Calories: 200
- Fat: 18g
- Carbohydrates: 4g
- Protein: 6g

GENEROUS FIERY TOMATO SALAD

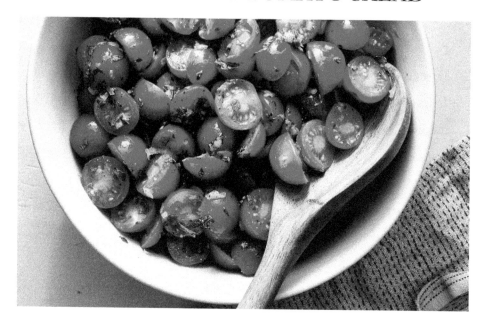

Serving: 4

Prep Time: 10 minutes

Cook Time: 25 minutes

Ingredients

- ½ cup scallions, chopped
- 1 pound cherry tomatoes
- 3 teaspoons olive oil
- Sea salt and freshly ground black pepper, to taste
- 1 tablespoon red wine vinegar

Directions

1. Season tomatoes with spices and oil

2. Heat your oven to 450-degree Fahrenheit

3. Take a baking sheet and spread the tomatoes

4. Bake for 15 minutes

5. Stir and turn the tomatoes

6. Then again, bake for 10 minutes

7. Take a bowl and mix the roasted tomatoes with all the remaining ingredients

8. Serve and enjoy!

Nutrition (Per Serving)

- Calories: 115
- Fat: 10.4g
- Carbohydrates: 5.4g
- Protein: 12g

EASY PORTOBELLO MUSHROOMS

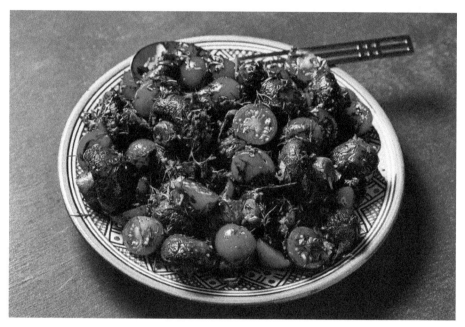

Serving: 4

Prep Time: 10 minutes

Cook Time: 10 minutes

Ingredients

- 12 cherry tomatoes
- 2 ounces scallions
- 4 portobello mushrooms
- 4 and ¼ ounces butter
- Salt and pepper to taste

Directions

1. Take a large skillet and melt butter over medium heat

2. Add mushrooms and Sauté for 3 minutes

3. Stir in cherry tomatoes and scallions

4. Sauté for 5 minutes

5. Season accordingly

6. Sauté until veggies are tender

7. Enjoy!

Nutrition (Per Serving)

- Calories: 154

- Fat: 10g

- Carbohydrates: 2g

- Protein: 7g

SIMPLE AVOCADO CAPRESE SALAD

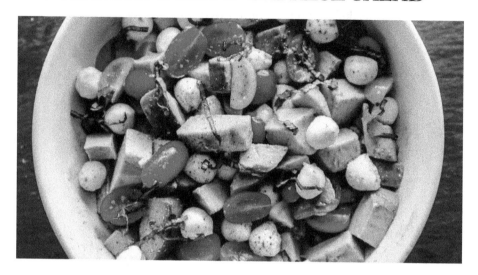

Serving: 6

Prep Time: 15 minutes

Cook Time: 29 minutes

Ingredients

- 2 avocados, cubed

- 1 cup cherry tomatoes, halved

- 8 ounces mozzarella balls, halved

- 2 tablespoons finely chopped fresh basil

- 2 tablespoons olive oil

- 2 tablespoons balsamic vinegar

- 1 tablespoon salt

- Fresh ground black pepper

Directions

1. Take a bowl and add the listed ingredients, toss them well until thoroughly mixed

2. Season with pepper according to your taste

3. Serve and enjoy!

Nutrition (Per Serving)

- Calories: 358
- Fat: 30g
- Carbohydrates: 9g
- Protein: 14g

LOVELY TURTLE SALAD

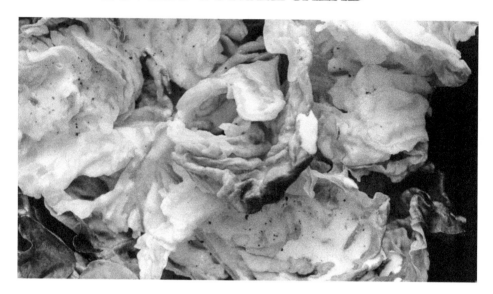

Serving: 2

Prep Time: 10 minutes

Cook Time: Nil

Ingredients

- 12 cups of rommain lettuce, chopped
- 1/3 cup of extra virgin olive oil
- 1/3 cup of fresh grated parmesan cheese
- 3 tablespoon of freshly squeezed lemon juice
- 1 and a ½ tablespoon of mayonnaise (Keto-Friendly)
- 1/3 teaspoon of garlic powder
- Freshly ground black pepper

Directions

1. Take a pan and place it over medium low heat

2. Add all of the ingredients and stir them until fully combined

3. Cook for about 5-10 minutes, making sure that the lid is on

4. Remove the lid and keep cooking until any excess liquid goes away

5. Once the rice is soft and creamy, enjoy!

Nutrition (Per Serving)

- Calories: 93
- Fat: 7g
- Carbohydrates: 4g
- Protein: 3g

GRILLED VEGGIE SALAD WITH FETA

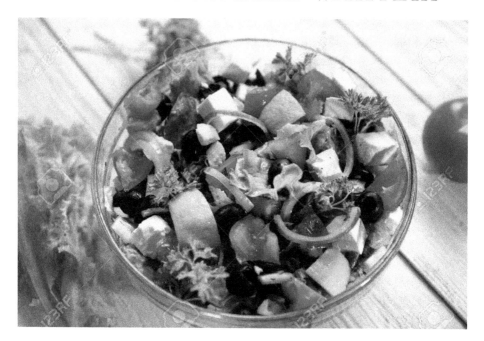

Serving: 4

Prep Time: 10 minutes

Cook Time: 10 minutes

Ingredients

- 3 grilling vegetables of your choice (e.g., eggplant, zucchini, and onions)

- $^1/2$ tsp oregano

- $^1/2$ cup of crumbled feta

- 2 tbsp of olive oil

- 1 tbsp of balsamic vinegar

Directions

1. In a grilling pan or in the broiler, cut the veggies into slices, season with oregano and salt/pepper, and cook until done for around 15 minutes.

2. Combine the olive oil and balsamic vinegar in a small cup or bowl to make a vinaigrette.

3. Drizzle the vinaigrette over the veggies and top with the crumbled feta pieces and serve

Nutrition (Per Serving)

- Calories: 191
- Fat: 14g
- Carbohydrates: 10g
- Protein: 9g

HEARTY VEGAN ZOODLES

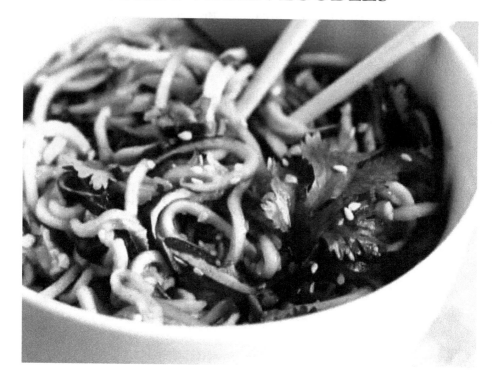

Serving: 2

Prep Time: 10 minutes

Cook Time: 10 minutes

Ingredients

- 4 small zucchinis spiralized into noodles
- $^1/2$ cup of diced onion
- $^1/2$ cup of red diced pepper
- 3 tbsp of vegetable stock
- $^3/4$ cup nutritional yeast

Directions

1. In a small pot over medium heat, combine the zoodles with the diced pepper and onions and vegetable stock until they have softened and the liquid has evaporated.

2. Toss in the nutritional yeast and stir well.

3. Serve in 1-2 bowls

Nutrition (Per Serving)

- Calories: 188
- Fat: 2g
- Carbohydrates: 23g
- Protein: 19g

GRILLED EGGPLANT ROLL

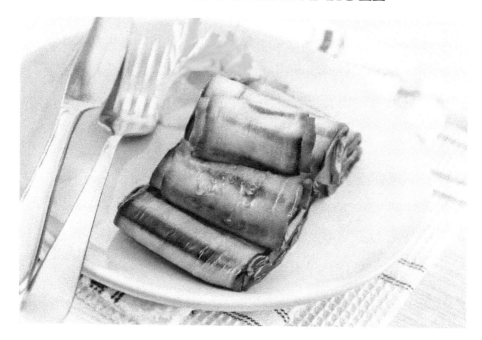

Serving: 4

Prep Time: 10 minutes

Cook Time: 8-10 minutes

Ingredients

- 1 eggplant aubergine, cut lengthwise into 7-8 thin slices with a sharp knife.
- 4 oz. of mozzarella
- 1 large tomato, sliced
- A bit of olive oil
- Salt to taste

Directions

1. Season the eggplant slices with salt and drizzle with olive oil.

2. In a grilling pan, grill the slices for 3 minutes on each side.

3. In a dish or board, arrange one tomato slice over each eggplant slice and top with mozzarella. Roll from left to right and secure with a toothpick.

4. Bake in the oven for 10 minutes at 375F/180 C or until cheese is melted.

5. Serve.

Nutrition (Per Serving)

- Calories: 59
- Fat: 3g
- Carbohydrates: 4g
- Protein: 3g

AVOCADO AND TOMATO BURRITOS

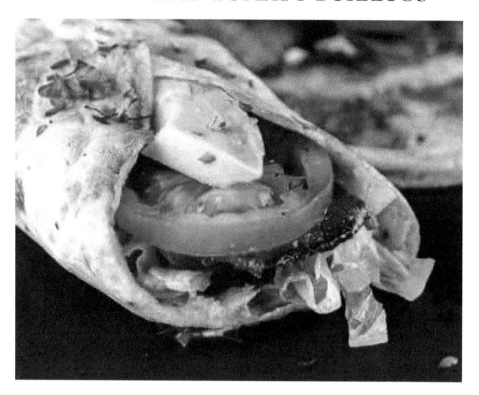

Serving: 4

Prep Time: 10 minutes

Cook Time: 2-5 minutes

Ingredients

- 2 cups cauli rice
- 6 low carb tortillas
- 2 cups sour cream sauce
- 1 $1/2$ cups tomato herb salsa
- 2 avocados, peeled, pitted, sliced

Directions

1. Pour the cauli rice into a bowl, sprinkle with a bit of water, and soften in the microwave for 2 minutes.

2. On the tortillas, spread the sour cream all over and distribute the salsa on top. Top with cauli rice and scatter the avocado evenly on top.

3. Fold and tuck the burritos and cut them into two

4. Serve and enjoy!

Nutrition (Per Serving)

- Calories: 303
- Fat: 25g
- Carbohydrates: 6g
- Protein: 8g

DARK CHOCOLATE FUDGE

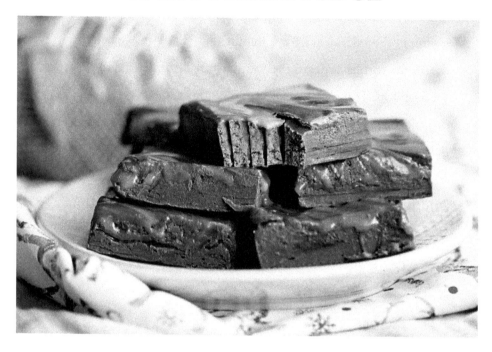

Serving: 4

Prep Time: 10 minutes

Cook Time: 20-25 minutes

Ingredients

- **1** cup dark chocolate, melted
- 4 large eggs
- 1 cup swerve sugar
- 1/2 cup melted butter
- 1/3 cup coconut flour

Directions

1. Preheat oven to 350 F and line a rectangular baking tray with parchment paper.

2. In a bowl, cream the eggs with swerving sugar until smooth. Add in melted chocolate, butter, and whisk until evenly combined.

3. Carefully fold in the coconut flour to incorporate and pour the mixture into the baking tray.

4. Bake for 20 minutes or until a toothpick inserted comes out clean. Remove from the oven and allow cooling in the tray.

5. Cut into squares and serve.

Nutrition (Per Serving)

- Calories: 491
- Fat: 45g
- Carbohydrates: 2.8g
- Protein: 13g

MOROCCAN ROASTED GREEN BEANS

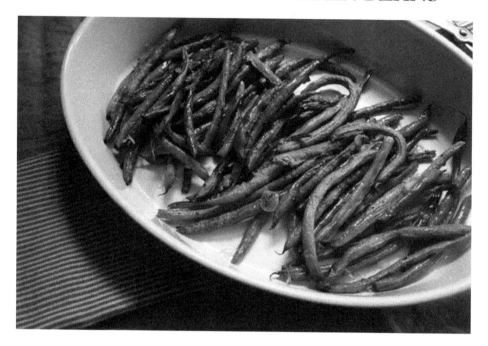

Serving: 4

Prep Time: 10 minutes

Cook Time: 15-20 minutes

Ingredients

- 5 oz green beans 1/2 tsp salt
- $^1/2$ tbsp Moroccan spice mix
- 1 $^1/2$ tbsp avocado oil

Directions

1. Turn on the oven, then set it to 400 degrees F and let it preheat.

2. Take a medium bowl, place green beans in it, add oil, salt, spice mix and

toss until well coated.

Spread green beans on a sheet pan and then bake for 15 minutes until roasted, stirring halfway.

Serve.

Nutrition (Per Serving)

- Calories: 103
- Fat: 0.8g
- Carbohydrates: 2g
- Protein: 2.3g

BALSAMIC GRILLED ZUCCHINI

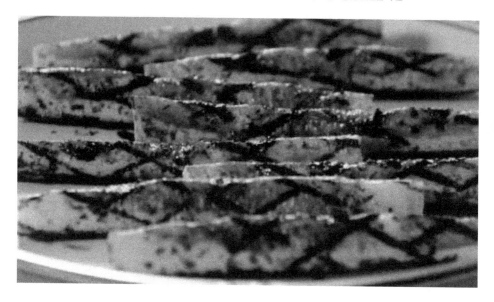

Serving: 4

Prep Time: 10 minutes

Cook Time: 10-15 minutes

Ingredients

- 1 zucchini, sliced lengthwise1/3 tsp garlic powder
- 1 tsp Italian seasoning
- 2 tbsp balsamic vinegar2 tsp avocado oil
- Seasoning:
- $^1/4$ tsp salt

Directions

1. Take a griddle pan, place it over medium-low heat, brush it with oil and let it preheat.

2. Meanwhile, brush zucchini slices with oil and then sprinkle with garlic powder, Italian seasoning, and salt.

3. Place zucchini slices on the griddle pan and cook for 2 to 3 minutes per side, then brush zucchini with vinegar and cook for another minute.

4. Serve and enjoy!

Nutrition (Per Serving)

- Calories: 76
- Fat: 5g
- Carbohydrates: 5g
- Protein: 6g

STIR FRIED ZUCCHINI AND GREEN BEANS

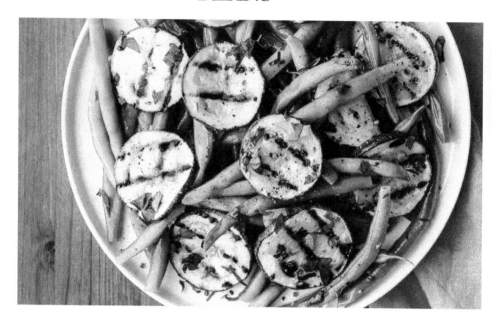

Serving: 4

Prep Time: 10 minutes

Cook Time: 10 minutes

Ingredients

- 3 tablespoons olive oil
- $^1/2$ small zucchini, thinly sliced
- $^1/2$ cup green beans, cut into small pieces
- Sea salt, to taste
- 2 tablespoons scallions, chopped
- 2 tablespoons lemon juice

Directions

1. Heat the olive oil in a nonstick skillet over medium heat.

2. Add and stir fry the zucchini, green beans, and salt for 9 minutes or until soft and crisp.

3. Remove them from the skillet to a plate. Garnish with chopped scallion and serve drizzled with lemon juice.

Nutrition (Per Serving)

- Calories: 137
- Fat: 13g
- Carbohydrates: 3g
- Protein: 1.2g

LIME AVOCADO ICE CREAM

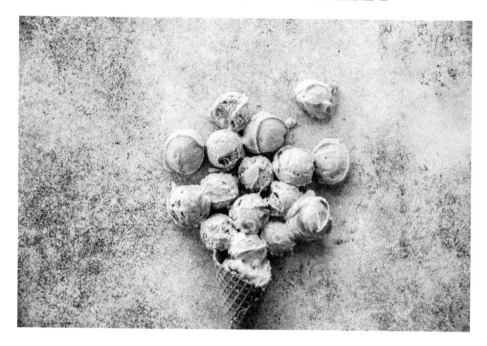

Serving: 4

Prep Time: 10 minutes

Cook Time: Nil

Ingredients

- 2 large avocados, pitted
- Juice and zest of 3 limes
- $^5/3$ cup erythritol
- 13/4 cups coconut cream
- $^1/4$ tsp vanilla extract

Directions

1. In a blender, combine avocado pulp, lime juice and zest, erythritol, coconut cream, and vanilla extract. Process until smooth.

2. Pour the mixture into an ice cream maker and freeze. When ready, remove and scoop the ice cream into bowls. Serve immediately.

Nutrition (Per Serving)

- Calories: 260
- Fat: 25g
- Carbohydrates: 4g
- Protein: 4g

COCONUT CAULIFLOWER RICE WITH GREEN ONIONS

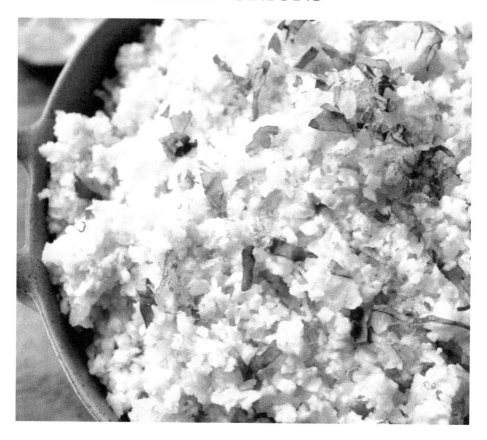

Serving: 4

Prep Time: 10 minutes

Cook Time: 5-10 minutes

Ingredients

- 3 oz grated cauliflower florets
- 2 green onions, sliced
- 2 tbsp shredded coconut, unsweetened
- 1 tbsp avocado oil
- 3 oz coconut milk, unsweetened

Directions

1. Take a medium skillet pan, place it over medium heat, add oil and when hot, add grated cauliflower and cook for 3 minutes until golden brown.

2. Add coconut, pour in milk, stir until mixed and cook for 1 to 2 minutes until hot and creamy.

3. Remove pan from heat, garnish cauliflower rice with green onions and then, serve.

Nutrition (Per Serving)

- Calories: 107
- Fat: 1.7g
- Carbohydrates: 2.1g
- Protein: 1.1g

BAKED BRUSSELS SPROUTS

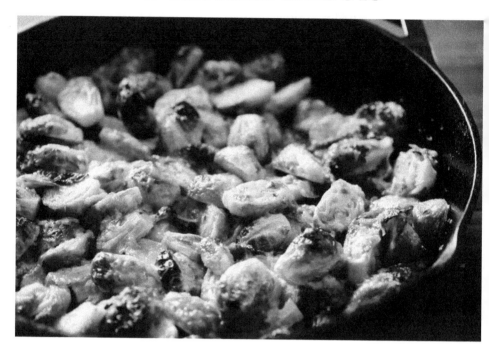

Serving: 4

Prep Time: 10 minutes

Cook Time: 20 minutes

Ingredients

- 1 pound Brussels sprouts, trimmed and halved
- 1 tablespoon avocado oil
- 2 garlic cloves, minced
- A pinch of salt and black peppers/4 cup cilantro, chopped

Directions

1. In a roasting pan, combine the sprouts with the oil and the other ingredients, toss and bake at 400 degrees F for 20 minutes.

2. Divide everything between plates and serve.

Nutrition (Per Serving)

- Calories: 100
- Fat: 3g
- Carbohydrates: 2g
- Protein: 6g

GARLIC TOUCHED BEANS

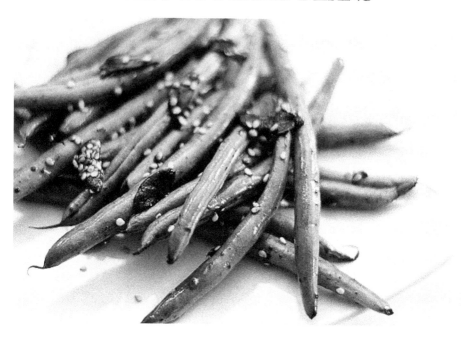

Serving: 4

Prep Time: 10 minutes

Cook Time: 5-10 minutes

Ingredients

- 1 lb green beans, trimmed
- 1 cup butter
- 2 cloves garlic, minced 1 cup toasted pine nuts

Directions

1. Boil a pot of water.

2. Add the green beans and cook until tender for 5 minutes.

3. Heat the butter in a large skillet over high heat. Add the garlic and pine nuts and sauté for 2 minutes or until the pine nuts are lightly browned.

4. Transfer the green beans to the skillet and turn until coated.

5. Serve!

Nutrition (Per Serving)

- Calories: 215
- Fat: 9g
- Carbohydrates: 7g
- Protein: 4g

KETO-FRIENDLY ROSEMARY FLAVORED GREEN BEANS

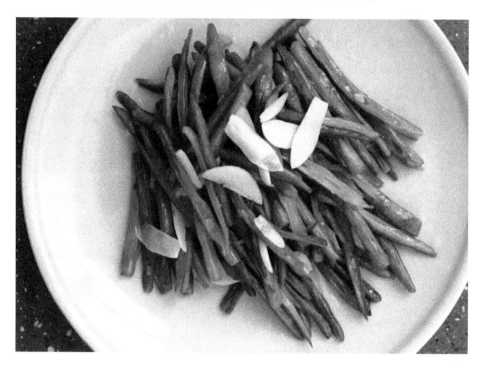

Serving: 4

Prep Time: 10 minutes

Cook Time:1 hour 30 minutes

<u>Ingredients</u>

- 1 pound green beans
- 1 tablespoon rosemary, minced
- 1 teaspoon fresh thyme, minced
- 2 tablespoons lemon juice
- 2 tablespoons water

Directions

1. Add all of the listed ingredients to your pot

2. Cook on LOW for about 3 hours, making sure to stir it from time to time

3. Once done, allow it to cool and serve!

Nutrition (Per Serving)

- Calories: 40
- Fat: 0g
- Carbohydrates: 9g
- Protein: 2g

CRAZY CARAMELIZED ONION

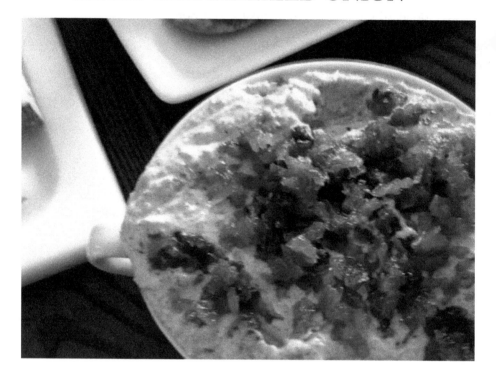

Serving: 4

Prep Time: 10 minutes

Cook Time:9-10 hours

Ingredients

- 6 onions, sliced
- 2 tablespoons oil
- ½ teaspoon salt

Directions

1. Add onions, oil, and salt to your Slow Cooker.

2. Close lid and cook on LOW for 8 hours.

3. Open the lid and keep simmering for 1-2 hours until any excess water has evaporated.

4. Serve and enjoy!

Nutrition (Per Serving)

- Calories: 126
- Fat: 15g
- Carbohydrates: 15g
- Protein: 2g

Tip: If you don't have a slow cooker, you may use an Iron-Cast Dutch Oven. The temperature is 200 Degrees F for LOW and 250 degrees F for HIGH

BROCCOLI CRUNCHIES

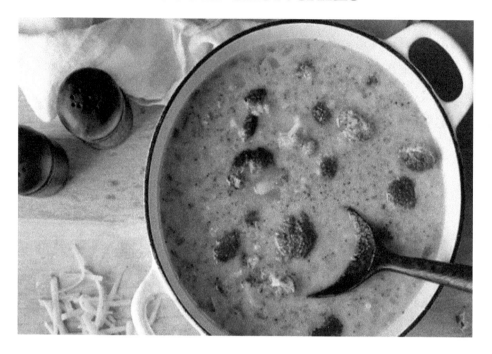

Serving: 4

Prep Time: 10 minutes

Cook Time:3 hours

Ingredients

- 2 cups broccoli florets + 1 small yellow onion, chopped
- 2 ounces cream of celery soup
- 2 tablespoons cheddar cheese, shredded
- ¼ teaspoon Worcestershire sauce
- ½ tablespoon butter

Directions

1. Add broccoli, cream, cheese, onion, cheddar to Slow Cooker

2. Stir and season with salt and pepper

3. Place lid and cook on LOW for 3 hours

4. Serve and enjoy!

Nutrition (Per Serving)

- Calories: 162

- Fat: 11g

- Carbohydrates: 11g

- Protein: 5g

Tip: If you don't have a slow cooker, you may use an Iron-Cast Dutch Oven. The temperature is 200 Degrees F for LOW and 250 degrees F for HIGH

THE EXTREMELY SLOW COOKED BRUSSELS

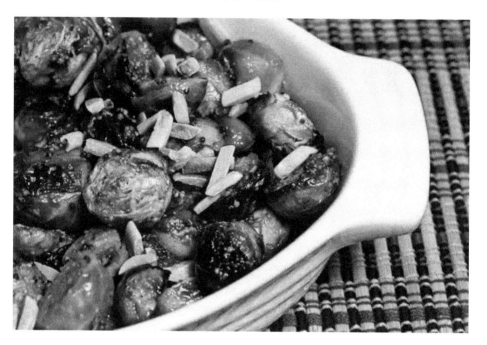

Serving: 4

Prep Time: 15 minutes

Cook Time:4 hours

Ingredients

- 1 pound Brussels sprouts, bottom trimmed and cut

- 1 tablespoon olive oil

- 1 -1/2 tablespoon Dijon mustard

- ¼ cup water

- ½ teaspoon dried tarragon

Directions

1. Add Brussels, salt, water, pepper, mustard to Slow Cooker

2. Add dried tarragon and stir

3. Place lid and cook on LOW for 5 hours until the Brussels are tender

4. Stir well and add Dijon over Brussels

5. Stir and enjoy!

Nutrition (Per Serving)

- Calories: 83

- Fat: 4g

- Carbohydrates: 11g

- Protein: 4g

Tip: If you don't have a slow cooker, you may use an Iron-Cast Dutch Oven. The temperature is 200 Degrees F for LOW and 250 degrees F for HIGH

A GREEN BEAN MIXTURE

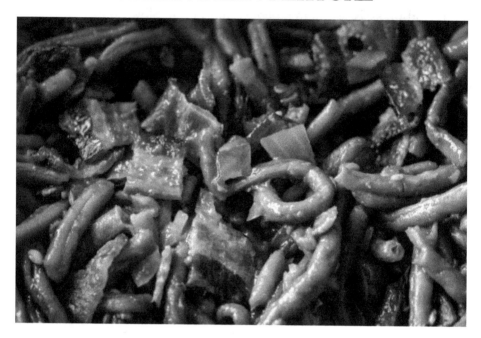

Serving: 2

Prep Time: 10 minutes

Cook Time:2 hours

Ingredients

- 4 cups green beans, trimmed

- 2 tablespoons butter, melted

- 1 tablespoon date paste

- Salt and pepper as needed

- ¼ teaspoon coconut aminos

Directions

1. Add green beans, date paste, pepper, salt, coconut aminos, and stir

2. Toss and place lid

3. Cook on LOW for 2 hours

4. Serve and enjoy!

Nutrition (Per Serving)

- Calories: 236
- Fat: 6g
- Carbohydrates: 10g
- Protein: 6g

CREAMY LEEKS PLATTER

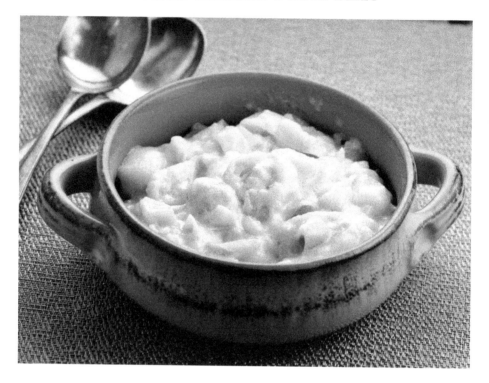

Serving: 6

Prep Time: 10 minutes

Cook Time: 25 minutes

Ingredients

- 1 and ½ pound leeks, trimmed and chopped into 4-inch pieces
- 2 ounces butter
- 1 cup coconut cream
- 3 and ½ ounces cheddar cheese
- Salt and pepper to taste

Directions

1. Preheat your oven to 400 degrees F

2. Take a skillet and place it over medium heat, add butter and let it heat up

3. Add leeks and Saute for 5 minutes

4. Spread leeks in greased baking dish

5. Boil cream in a saucepan and lower heat to low

6. Stir in cheese, salt, and pepper

7. Pour sauce over leeks

8. Bake for 15-20 minutes and serve warm

9. Enjoy!

Nutrition (Per Serving)

- Calories: 204

- Fat: 15g

- Carbohydrates: 9g

- Protein: 7g

SUCCULENT CHEESY CAULIFLOWERS

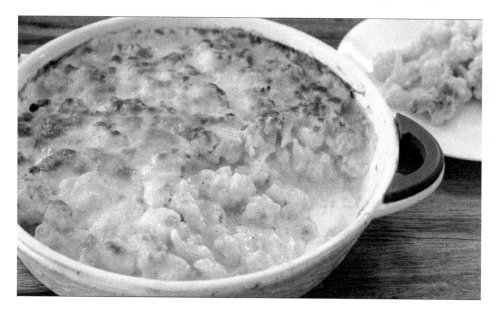

Serving: 3

Prep Time: 10 minutes

Cook Time: 25 minutes

Ingredients

- 1 cauliflower head
- ¼ cup butter, cut into small pieces
- 1 teaspoon Keto-Friendly Mayo
- 1 tablespoon Keto-Friendly Mustard
- ½ cup parmesan cheese, grated

Directions

1. Preheat your oven to 390 degrees F

2. Add mayo and mustard in a bowl

3. Add cauliflower to mayo mix and toss

4. Spread cauliflower in a baking dish and top with butter

5. Sprinkle cheese on top

6. Bake for 25 minutes

7. Serve and enjoy!

Nutrition (Per Serving)

- Calories: 228

- Fat: 20g

- Carbohydrates: 6g

- Protein: 3g

CREAMY CAULI MUSHROOM RISOTTO

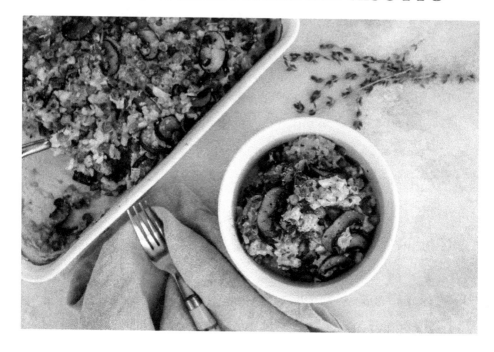

Serving: 4

Prep Time: 10 minutes

Cook Time: 20 minutes

Ingredients

- 1 cup vegetable stock
- 1 head of cauliflower, grated
- 9 ounces mushroom, chopped
- 2 tablespoons butter
- 1 cup coconut cream

Directions

1. Take a saucepan and pour the stock into it

2. Bring it to boil and set it aside

3. Then take a skillet and melt butter over medium heat

4. Add mushroom to sauté until it turns into golden brown

5. Stir in a stock and grated cauliflower

6. Bring the mixture to a simmer and add cream

7. Cook until liquid is reduced and cauliflower is aldente

8. Serve warm and enjoy!

Nutrition (Per Serving)

- Calories: 186

- Fat: 16.5g

- Carbohydrates: 6.7g

- Protein: 2.8g

CELERY SAUTÉ

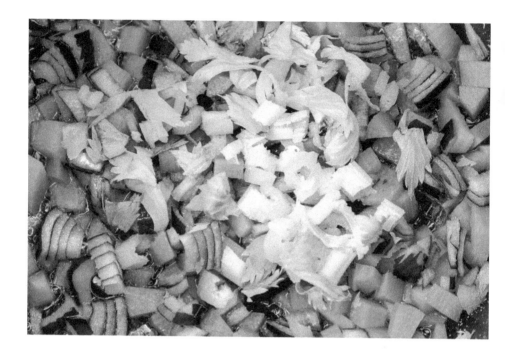

Preparation time: 10 minutes

Cooking time: 20 minutes

Servings: 4

Ingredients:

- 2 tablespoons olive oil
- 3 celery stalks, roughly chopped
- 2 shallots, chopped
- ¼ cup veggie stock
- 1 tablespoon parmesan, grated
- A pinch of salt and black pepper

Directions:

1. Heat up a pan with the oil over medium-high heat, add the shallots and sauté for 3 minutes.

2. Add the celery and the other ingredients, toss, cook everything over medium heat for 12 minutes more, divide between plates and serve.

Nutrition (Per Serving)

- Calories 193
- Fat 14
- Fiber 3
- Carbs 6
- Protein 5

BAKED TOMATO MIX

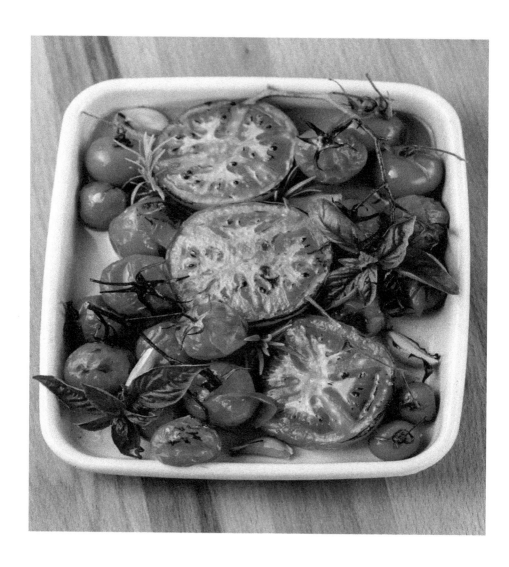

Preparation time: 10 minutes

Cooking time: 25 minutes

Servings: 4

Ingredients:

- 1 pound tomatoes, cut into wedges
- 1 tablespoon balsamic vinegar
- 2 tablespoons olive oil
- A pinch of salt and black pepper
- 1 tablespoon basil, chopped

Directions:

1. Spread the tomatoes on a baking sheet lined with parchment paper, add the vinegar and the other ingredients, toss gently, and cook at 400 degrees F for 25 minutes.
2. Divide between plates and serve hot as a side dish.

Nutrition (Per Serving)

- Calories 55
- Fat 1
- Fiber 1
- Carbs 0.5
- Protein 7

CHILI MUSTARD GREENS

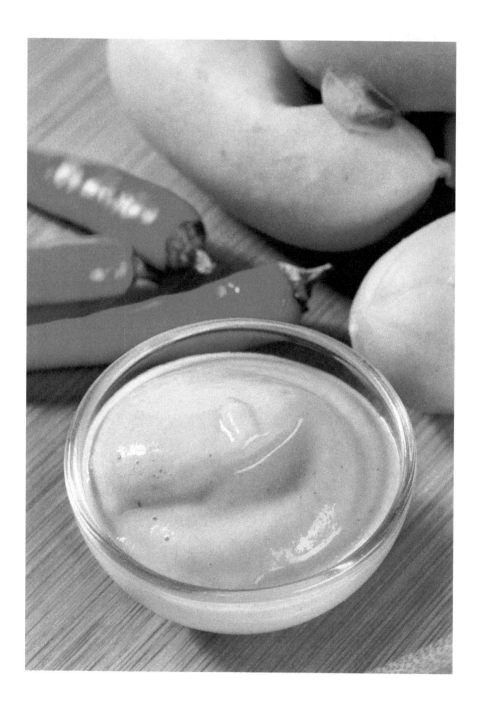

Preparation time: 10 minutes

Cooking time: 15 minutes

Servings: 4

Ingredients:

- 1 pound mustard greens
- 1 teaspoon chili powder
- 2 tablespoons olive oil
- 3 garlic cloves, minced
- ½ cup veggie stock
- A pinch of salt and black pepper
- 1 tablespoon red pepper flakes, crushed
- 1 tablespoon chives, chopped

Directions:

1. Heat up a pan with the oil over medium heat, add the garlic and sauté for 2minutes.
2. Add the mustard greens and the other ingredients, toss, bring to a simmer and cook over medium heat for 13 minutes more.
3. Divide the mix between plates and serve as a side dish.

Nutrition (Per Serving)

- Calories 143
- Fat 3
- Fiber 4
- Carbs 3
- Protein 4.6

MINTY ZUCCHINIS

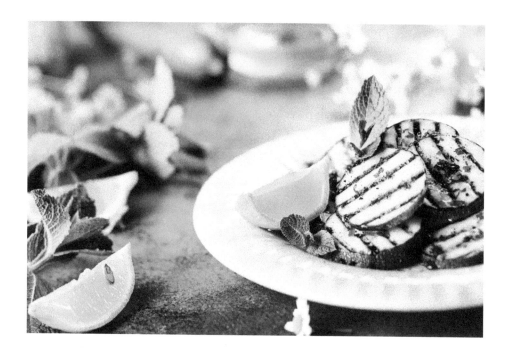

Preparation time: 10 minutes
Cooking time: 15 minutes
Servings: 4

Ingredients:

- 1 pound zucchinis, sliced
- 1 tablespoon olive oil
- 2 garlic cloves, minced
- 1 tablespoon mint, chopped
- A pinch of salt and black pepper
- ¼ cup veggie stock

Directions:

1. Heat up a pan with the oil over medium high heat, add the garlic and sauté for 2 minutes.

2. Add the zucchinis and the other ingredients, toss, cook everything for 10 minutes more, divide between plates and serve as a side dish.

Nutrition (Per Serving)

- Calories 70
- Fat 1
- Fiber 1
- Carbs 0.4
- Protein 6

MEASUREMENTS & CONVERSIONS

	US STANDARD	US STANDARD (OUNCES)	METRIC (APPROXIMATE)
VOLUME EQUIVALENTS (LIQUID)	2 tablespoon	1 fl. oz.	30 mL
	1/4 cup	2 fl. oz.	60 mL
	1/2 cup	4 fl. oz.	120 mL
	1 cup	8 fl. oz.	240 mL
	1 1/2 cup	12 fl. oz.	355 mL
	2 cups or 1 pint	16 fl. oz.	475 mL
VOLUME EQUIVALENTS DRY	1/4 teaspoon		1 mL
	1/2 teaspoon		2 mL
	1 teaspoon		5 mL
	1 tablespoon		15 mL
	1/4 cup		59 mL
	1/3 cup		79 mL
	1/2 cup		118 mL
	2/3 cup		156 mL
	3/4 cup		177 mL
	1 cup		235 mL
	2 cups or 1 pint		475 mL
	3 cup		700 mL
	4 cups or 1 quart		1 L
WEIGHT EQUIVALENTS	1/2 ounce		15 g
	1 ounce		30 g
	2 ounces		60 g
	4 ounces		115 g
	8 ounces		225 g
	12 ounces		340 g
	16 ounces or 1 pound		455 g

	FAHRENHEIT (F)	CELSIUS (C) (APPROXIMATE)
OVEN TEMPERATURES	250 °F	120 °C
	300 °F	150 °C
	325 °F	180 °C
	375 °F	190 °C
	400 °F	200 °C
	425 °F	220 °C
	450 °F	230 °C

CPSIA information can be obtained
at www.ICGtesting.com
Printed in the USA
LVHW082041220621
690870LV00008B/356